MAXIMIZE EXERCISE WORKOUTS THROUGH JUICING

Take Exercising to the Next Level with Proper Liquid Nutrition

RON KNESS

Contents

Introduction

Juicing is a great way to get your body pumped and primed for a lengthy workout session. When you juice, you cram loads of essential nutrients into one glass that will power your workout and improve your results.

Besides the important health benefits, key plant nutrients give you energy so you perform at your best in your workouts and get the most out of your exercise efforts.

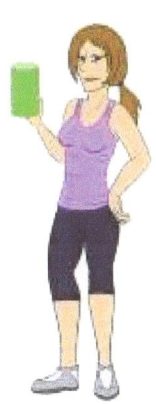

Because a lot of us don't like eating whole fruit and vegetables, we struggle to get our fill of the essential micronutrients.

Micronutrients are gems of nature for our bodies and minds. Without them, our bodies aren't ready for a workout.

Juicing is a fantastic and tasty way of stuffing yourself with the right amount of nutrients at the right time in a convenient manner.

Get ready to learn all about the ultimate warriors of the juicing world. You're going to discover the nutrients, the fruit, and vegetables that enhance your workout, boost your staying power, and help you take your exercise regimen to the next level.

Let's go!

Role of Nutrition in Exercising

Perhaps you already know that **what** you eat is really important. But what you're perhaps looking to learn is why **when** you eat is so important too - especially if you exercise.

If you drink the right nutrient-stuffed juice an hour or two before exercise and follow it up with another an hour or two after your exercise, you're pretty much meeting all your workout nutrition needs. You don't really need anything else.

However, it can also depend on what you're looking to get out of your workout. If, for example you're an endurance athlete who trains every day for high-level competition, you'll need more carbs and calories than the average person who exercises. You also need more protein.

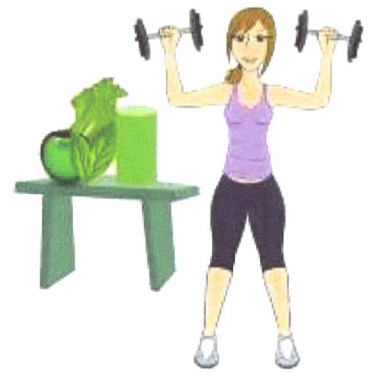

On the other hand, maybe you're training as a bodybuilder who lifts weights in order to seriously grow muscles. Because you're looking to gain more weight, you'll need more protein and carbs. Alternatively, you may be looking to get ready for a fitness competition, in which case your cab intake should be reduced.

It also comes down to your body type. If you have an **ectomorph**, you'll probably be looking to gain more muscle. If you have a **mesomorph**, you'll probably be looking to optimize your physique.

If you have an **endomorph**, you'll probably be looking to lose body fat.

However, it all comes down to the same thing: We all need nutrients to power us through a workout, and juicing them is just plain easier and faster than eating them.

PRE-WORKOUT NUTRITION

What and **when** we eat before we workout can often make a huge different to not only your performance, but also the way you recover.

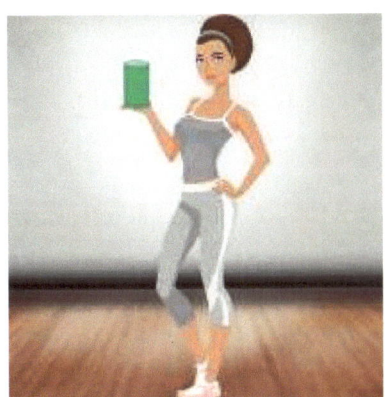

You need to eat or drink about two to three hours before a workout with nutrients that will:

- Sustain your energy

- Boost your performance

- Keep you nicely hydrated

- Preserve your muscle mass

- Speed up your recovery time

CARBOHYDRATES

Carbs are important because consuming these before exercise will fuel your training, giving you lots of energy, and they will also help you recover.

Many people say that you only need carbs if you're going to be engaged in a lengthy workout session, but that's just not true.

Let's say you want to do a shorter workout, but you want it to be high-intensity. You need lots of energy, right?

Unless your idea of exercise is to go for a stroll in the park and feed the birds, you're going to need to stock up on carbs.

Carbs also retain muscle and liver glycogen, which is important because it is this that tells your brain you have been well fed and don't need any more food during your workout. The last thing you want is to get hungry after 30 minutes. Carbs also stimulate the production of insulin, which prevents protein breakdown. Moreover, this is why you absolutely need to start juicing and stop drinking sugary energy drinks.

FATS

Healthy fats are another essential macronutrient that you need.

The funny thing about fats is that they don't improve your performance - but they don't really weaken it either. What they do is slow down digestion, which keeps your body on an even keel in terms of its insulin and blood glucose levels. They also provide you with some micronutrients, too.

PROTEIN

You can drink some of your juice during exercise, and it should be high protein because protein helps to prevent muscle breakdown, which leads to a better recovery post-workout. It also ensures that you adapt better to training as you progress, which means that you are better able to power your way through your workout.

You don't need a massive amount of protein in your juice; just a small amount is enough to prevent protein breakdown. If you like exercising on an empty stomach, then you don't need any more than around 15 grams of protein during training.

Athletes who do punishing training bouts need more protein, as does anyone who is looking to gain a significant amount of mass.

MICRONUTRIENTS

Lots of people know how to get their macronutrients - such as fats, carbs and protein - but they don't always stop to think about the role that vitamins and minerals (micronutrients) play in helping them power their way through a workout.

- ✓ Micronutrients play a really key role in energy production
- ✓ They also help to strengthen bones, boost your immune system, instigate hemoglobin synthesis, and protect you against oxidative damage
- ✓ Vitamins and minerals also repair muscle tissue that has been damaged during exercise.

You have to remember that workout stresses numerous metabolic pathways, and if we are to stay on top of these pathways and aid their recovery, we need micronutrients.

It's the same as when a car breaks down on a highway - it needs assistance from an auto repair company, otherwise, it's just dead on its wheels.

Moreover, when we exercise more and more, we experience muscle biochemical adaptations. To cope with these changes, we need even more micronutrients.

Even routine exercise can lead to a loss of too many micronutrients. These leaves you feeling fatigued. It doesn't help you to finish off a workout. Your body takes ages to repair, and you may even come away with a few injuries.

The key nutrients that athletes include in their diets are:

- Calcium
- Vitamin B
- Vitamin C
- Vitamin D
- Vitamin E
- Iron
- Magnesium

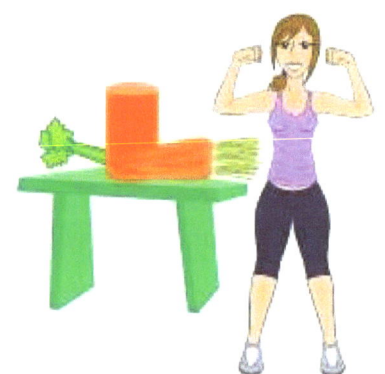

And the best place to get more micronutrients?

From juicing, of course.

Why?

Juicing is easy, and convenient, what is more convenient than drinking your nutrients?

An 8-ounce vegetable juice blend is like eating 2 large salads without the dressing.

It's portable, so you can easily drink them on your way to the gym, and on the drive home!

Key Nutrients That Power Your Workout

B-VITAMINS

If you've been working out for almost an hour but you find yourself running out of steam towards the end, the problem could be that you're lacking in B vitamins.

B Vitamins include:

- Thiamin
- Riboflavin
- Vitamin B-6
- Folate
- Vitamin B-12

If you've ever bought an energy drink, you may have noticed that they contain nutrients from the B-vitamin family, including thiamin, B12, riboflavin, and many others. The reason for this is that B-vitamins give you a burst of energy. They're essential for the conversion of food into fuel. Essential really means essential because without them you will have little energy. The body uses the B-vitamins to convert sugar and protein into fuel so athletes get as many of them as they can.

According to experts from the Department of Nutrition at Arizona State University which posted on MedlinePlus Health Information, B-vitamins, which include thiamin, riboflavin, and vitamin B-6) are necessary for energy-producing pathways in the body. Additionally, folate and vitamin B-12 are necessary to synthesize new red blood cells and to repair damaged cells.

Active individuals with a B-vitamin deficit may experience diminished performance during high intensity workouts.

The **major difference between vitamin B from juices made at home and that energy drink** is the latter is filled with other bad ingredients that have landed people in the emergency room, but your juice only has fresh produce and nutrients - **Winning!**

CALCIUM

You've probably heard all about calcium and how it strengthens the bones and you probably realize that a super strong skeleton is fundamental if you're going to working out, right?

Therefore, it makes sense that calcium should be one of the key nutrients that power your workouts. It increases your bone density, which ensures that your skeleton is strong enough for a great workout.

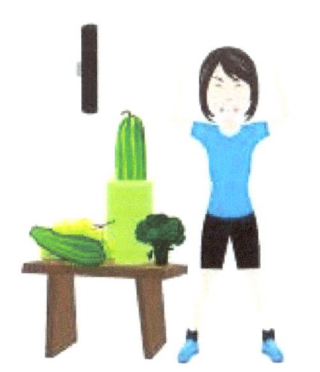

Milk is not the only source of calcium, you can get it from vegetables, and it's a better source since vegetables have no fat, no cholesterol, and they are low in calories.

VITAMIN C

Did you know that if you work out in colder climates, you could suffer from exercise-induced asthma? Not to raise any alarm bells, but that chesty cough you've been battling with these past few months could in fact be asthma.

In addition, it could be that your immune system is not as healthy as you might think. This can be resolved with Vitamin C, which naturally occurs in citrus fruits and various vegetables, and can boost your immunity, protect your cells from free radicals, and a slew of other functions that builds a better body that is powered for exercise.

Moreover, the more vitamin C you have, the easier it is to avoid contracting the flu and the common cold.

VITAMIN D

We all need vitamin D, right? Vitamin D comes from the sun and it makes us feel amazing. For many of us, the more sun we have the better we feel. It just imbues us with positivity and motivation. Vitamin D boosts your mood, and in this way, it can increase your determination to make it through a workout like a beast.

However, your mood alone will not get you through all the obstacles; you need something more. You need power, too. You don't need to go searching too far, though, because according to Science Daily vitamin D has been studied and found to be linked with increased muscle efficiency.

It may also be fantastic at tightening up your skeletal muscle function. These are some pretty awesome findings.

VITAMIN E

When we're sick, we don't really feel like doing anything. We're just not at our best. We don't feel like filing all those documents at work, going out on that date tonight ... and we especially don't feel in the mood for powering through the workout.

It's funny, but it always seems as though some people are more susceptible to getting sick than others are. Perhaps it's you that always seems to be sick, while your friends are constantly motoring through their workout like a warrior.

The reason for this could be that you deficient in vitamin E. Consuming more vitamin E can lower your risk of infection. It can make you almost immune to the common cold, the flu, and can slash your risk of developing pneumonia by almost 70%.

IRON

Popeye loved his spinach because he knew it contained lots of iron that would power his way through a workout. His nemesis Bluto must have loved the dark leafy green even more, because he was even bigger!

Iron is one of the key nutrients you need a lot more of if you want to own your workouts and fight fatigue; it's also integral in the metabolizing proteins, hemoglobin production, and red blood cell health.

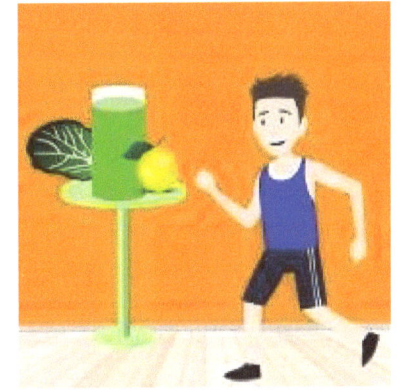

Here is some quick science:

- Each time you work out for an hour, your body loses around 5.6% of iron. That's quite significant.

- What happens next is your red blood cells struggle to carry as much oxygen to your muscles.

- Moreover, when your muscles don't get enough oxygen, you quickly get fatigued and may not be able to complete your workout.

MAGNESIUM

Magnesium is an absolute powerhouse mineral that top athletes make a priority. Magnesium is actually composed of over 300 enzymes that aid energy metabolism.

It also helps to strengthen your bones, which as previously mentioned is vital for your workout. As well as having a strong skeleton, you always need to avoid stress fractures as much as possible, and magnesium will help you do just that.

In addition, because you lose a lot of magnesium through sweat, you really need to consume as much of it as possible to replenish the supply lost in your workouts.

POTASSIUM

No doubt, you've seen tennis players munching away on bananas during a break in play. This is because bananas are super rich in potassium, a vital nutrient that speeds up recovery and nips cramps in the bud.

Juicing for Micronutrients: Key Ingredients

Now that you know that what key micronutrients you need to power your workout, you're probably wondering about the best sources for these, here are your best fruit and vegetable sources that will provide you with much needed nutrition through power juicing.

Calcium

Calcium is found in quite a few great juicing vegetables, which means that you get to choose what works for you.

- **Kale** is incredibly rich in calcium, and is one of the most 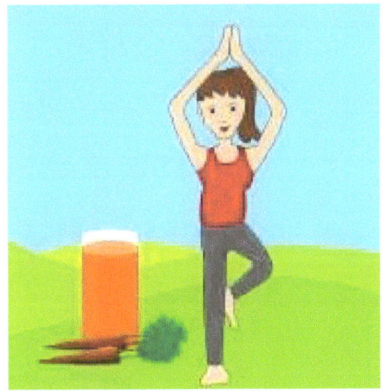 popular juicing vegetables, making up the bulk of the very healthy green juice. It delivers 139mg of calcium per every 100g serving. The best thing is that it's easily absorbed by the body.

- **Broccoli** is another great vegetable for juicing that is a fantastic source of calcium, and a single cup serving returns around 74mg.

- **Spinach** is a good leafy green alternative to kale (or you can juice both together), that contains around 145mg of calcium for every 100g serving. Yes, that's even better than kale.

- **Kelp** is also another fantastic source of calcium; a single cup serving returns around 136mg of this essential nutrient.

Vitamin C

Vitamin C could easily turn out to be your favorite micronutrient because so many tasty fruits and vegetables are loaded with it.

- The exotic and super delicious **guavas** always add a kick to juices, and a 100g serving contains a whopping 228mg of vitamin C.

- **Kiwifruit** might be something of an acquired taste, but if you love it, you're going to love the fact that a 100g serving contains 92mg of vitamin C.

- **Strawberries** are also rich in vitamin C, with a 100g serving containing almost 60mg of the nutrient.

- Then there are the zesty **citrus fruits**, ideal for juicing and especially to enhance the flavor of vegetable juices. **Lemons, limes, grapefruits** give you around 53mg of vitamin C per fruit.

- **Apples** contain lots of vitamin C, as do **tomatoes, kale,** and **broccoli**.

Vitamin E

- **Avocados** don't juice well, however they can be blended and mixed in with juice for a half and half smoothie juice blend. A 100g serving is enough to return 2.2mg of the often hard-to-get-hold-of vitamin E.

- **Sunflower seeds are loaded with vitamin E,** 36mg for every 100g serving and they are a great source of healthy fats. You can sprinkle these on top of your juice or grind them up and stir into a ready-made juice.

- **Broccoli** is also a good source of vitamin E, with a 100g serving delivering 1.5mg to your body and broccoli juices great.

- **Squash** and **pumpkin** return around 1.3mg each per 100g serving, while **blackberries** are 8% vitamin E, **peaches** are 7%, and **raspberries** are 5%.

Iron

- You can look to **spinach** for your iron intake. This dark leafy green vegetable delivers 3.57mg of iron per ever 100g serving.

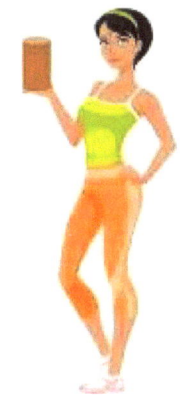

- **Asparagus** is another good source, and returns 2.14mg of iron for every 100g serving.
- Berries are really good sources, too: **elderberries** are 13% iron, while **raspberries** are 9% and **blackberries** are 5%.
- If you want to try something a little bit different in your juice, how about **coconut**? A 100g serving contains 3.32mg of iron.

Potassium

Many fruits and vegetables are rich in potassium.

- **Guavas**, which contain 417mg per 100g serving.
- **Bananas** are well known for their potassium content, and they return 358mg per 100g serving. Bananas don't juice, but they blend so you can stir them into your finished juices.
- **Spinach** juices great and has 167mg per I cup, if you juice 3 cups you are getting more than 15% of the daily recommended value of potassium.
- **Passion fruit** should be on your grocery list too, as this silky fruit contains 348mg per 100g serving.
- **Apricots** are also a good source of potassium, with every 100g serving returning 259mg.
- **Pomegranates** contain 236mg per 100g serving, while **cherries** deliver 222mg to your body.

Magnesium

- All dark leafy greens, including **Kale, spinach, chard, and collard greens** are high in magnesium.
- **Cherries, coconut, papaya, bananas, watermelon, and peaches** are your best fruit choices for magnesium intake.

Vitamin D

There are many choices in great juicing fruits and vegetables for vitamin D.

- **Kale** is one of the best sources of vitamin D supplying 6,693 IU per cup
- **Spinach** comes in second with 2,813 IU per cup
- **Swiss chard** has 2,202 IU per cup
- You can also get it from, **kohlrabi, asparagus, bitter melon** including the leafy tops, **broccoli, cauliflower, zucchini** and **cucumber**
- **Grapefruits** with 2,830 IU per fruit
- **Mangoes** 1,785 IU per 1 cup
- **Papaya** with 1,492 IU per 1 small fruit

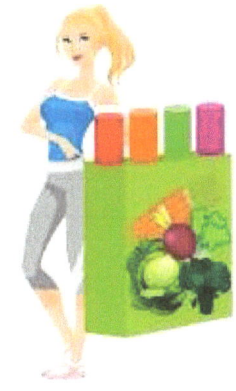

- **Tomatoes**, with 1,025 IU per 1 medium tomato
- **Watermelon** has 865 IU per 1 cup diced
- Other fruits include, **cranberries, gooseberries, grapes, passionfruit, and peaches**

B-Vitamins

Riboflavin

Vegetable sources include **beet Greens, Asparagus, spinach, collard greens, Dandelion Greens** and other **dark green leafy vegetables, peppers, Brussels sprouts, Asparagus and Broccoli**.

Fresh fruit sources include **blueberries, apples, passion fruit,** and **avocado**. When it comes to fruit, many offer higher counts in dried form which is not appropriate for juicing, plus dried fruit is not your best choice in any case, since it is much higher in sugar than fresh fruit.

Folate

Vegetable sources include **leafy greens** such as **spinach** and **turnip greens**

Fruit sources include **oranges** with the most at about 50 mcg per fruit and one large glass of orange juice providing even more. Other folate-rich fruits include **grapes, banana, cantaloupe, papaya, grapefruit,** and **strawberries**.

Vitamin B6

Vegetable sources include leafy green vegetables: **spinach, kale, greens,** and **broccoli.**

Fruit sources include **bananas.**

The Power of Beets

This chapter is dedicated to beets, which can go a long way to power your workouts and improve your overall performance.

BEETS CONTAIN A WEALTH OF NUTRIENTS

Yes, beets contain a wide variety of healthy nutrients, including:

- Beets are a unique source of phytonutrients called betalains that have anti- antioxidant, anti-inflammatory, and detoxification properties.
- Beetroots are rich in inorganic nitrates, which are compounds that encourage the signaling molecule Nitric Oxide to take action.
- Folate - 34% DRI/DV per 1 cup
- Manganese - 28% DRI/DV per 1 cup
- Potassium - 15% DRI/DV per 1 cup
- Copper - 14% DRI/DV per 1 cup
- Fiber - 14% DRI/DV per 1 cup
- Magnesium - 10% DRI/DV per 1 cup
- Phosphorus - 9% DRI/DV per 1 cup
- Vitamin C - 8% DRI/DV per 1 cup
- Iron - 7% DRI/DV per 1 cup
- Vitamin B6 - 6% DRI/DV per 1 cup

BENEFITS

✓ Beetroots are so good for you as they improve brain functioning, which is what you need when the tough gets going down at the gym. Many people underestimate the power of mental resilience, but you should never underestimate it.

✓ Beets also promote stronger bones, and as we all know a super strong skeleton is essential for a good workout.

✓ Beets also boost your immune system lowering your chances of getting sick and missing days at the gym.

Yet people keep on ignoring these purple veggies whenever they do their weekly shop. As a matter of fact, beetroots must be one of the most overlooked veggies in America. It's amazing how people who see these colorful vegetables screaming at them "pick me! pick me!" but opt for lettuce again, as usual.

Get out of your comfort zone, and get into juicing beetroots. Elite athletes all around the world use them, and they'll tell you that beets are the vegetables that give them the edge over their competitors.

THE SCIENCE BEHIND BEETS

Beetroots are rich in inorganic nitrates, which are compounds that encourage the signaling molecule Nitric Oxide to take action.

NO is made in our bodies but we don't always produce very much of it. To produce more of it, we need to eat food that is rich in nitrate - such as beets.

NO improves the strength of our skeleton, and increases the amount of oxygen that is sent to our brain.

WHY JUICE BEETS?

According to research, drinking around 500ml of beetroot juice per day can keep us feeling more energetic. In fact, drinking beet juice can keep us going in the gym for 15% more time than we normally would.

Many people think that juicing just takes up too much time, and it's too messy. However when you have the right equipment and plan ahead, it is much easier than you think.

If you have the time to make yourself some juice in the morning before a workout, this is something you should definitely think about doing.

Alternatives include beet powder and concentrated juices, but these are often filled with artificial substances, too much sugar, and not enough fiber or nutrients - basically, they don't have the same amount of good stuff as beet juice does.

How Much Do You Need

As previously stated, 500ml of beet juice per day is enough to increase our staying power by around 15%. This equates to 2 cups. However, go ahead find a dose that works for you, if 250ml of beet juice a day increases your staying power by 10%, then go for it.

Some athletes drink more than 600ml, but again it's all about how much you can handle.

Cooked Or Raw

Research in the past has shown that cooking beetroots can reduce the nitrates content - which is not what we really want. For this reason, it's best to juice with raw beets only.

Drink It Slow

It takes a while for the nitrates in beets to be ingested, and used by your body. They enter our mouth, where they are manipulated by saliva. This takes a bit of time, so if you clean your teeth not long after eating (and many people do this after eating beets in order to get rid of the purple color) you will only be washing all the beneficial nitrates out of your mouth. Drink slowly for better conversion rates.

Does It Work For Everyone?

Beet juice works for many people, many boost their workouts, but like with anything, our body's all respond in different ways.

What works for some might not work for others. The only really accurate way you can find out is by giving it a go. Other high nitrate vegetables include spinach and kale.

10 Workout Boosting Juice Recipes

Here are some great juicing recipes to power your workouts. These recipes pack a lot of punch and they will fuel your pre and post-workout routines.

Preparation of these juices will depend on your juicer model, as they are all different in requirements for cutting, speed settings and order in which to juice.

Get juicing!

MAGNESIUM MAGIC

Too many of us don't get enough magnesium, yet this micronutrient plays an essential role in a solid workout. If you're looking to find a way of sneaking more of this mineral into your diet, this represents a fantastic way to do so.

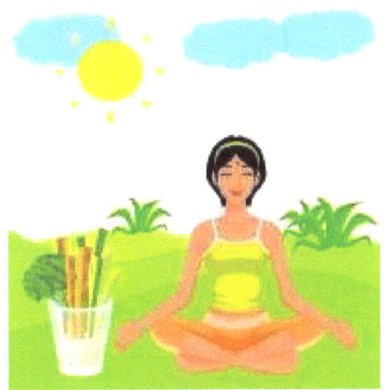

Ingredients:

- Large Handful Of Parsley
- 3 leaves of chard
- 1 Cup Watermelon
- 4 carrots
- 1 Peach
- 2 Celery Stalks Including The Leafy Tops
- 1 Lemon

DYNAMITE BLEND

Stop reaching for a sports drink after your exercise, and start making this antioxidant-and vitamin C rich juice instead. It's super rich in all your essential vitamins and minerals.

Ingredients:

- 1 Orange
- 2 Kale Leaves (or collard greens leaves)
- 1 Green Apple
- 1 Lemon
- 1 Lime
- 4 Broccoli Florets (including stems and leaves)

REPAIR AND RECOVERY

This is nature's best antidote for aiding recovery so that you can go again soon. It helps to repair muscle and tissue damage and makes your body tougher over the long-term.

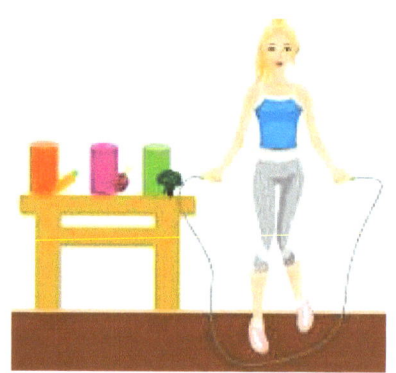

Ingredients:

- 1 Green Apple
- ½ Cup Strawberries
- ½ Pound Of Organic Tart Cherries
- 2 Celery Stalks
- 4 Kale Leaves
- ½ Cucumber
- ½ Lemon

THE RED RESURRECTOR

Tomato juice is super rich in electrolytes, and ideal for maintaining proper hydration during and before a workout. Tomatoes also have many other health benefits and essential antioxidants to prevent chronic disease.

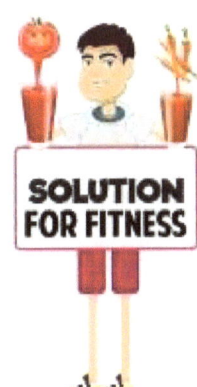

This juice includes an added boost from coconut water, which is naturally rich in electrolytes, so you can skip the sports drink and get your energy from juice instead.

Ingredients:

- 1 Lemon
- 5 Medium Carrots
- 2 Tomatoes
- 1 Cucumber (super hydration)
- Handful Of Cilantro
- 1/ Cup Of Coconut Water

BEET POWER JUICE

Ingredients:

- 3 carrots
- 3 kale leaves
- 1 Beet Including Leafy Tops
- 1" Piece of Fresh Ginger

- 1 Garlic Clove
- 1 Lime
- ½ Grapefruit

POST WORKOUT BLISS JUICE

Another great all natural post-workout recovery blend.

Ingredients:

- 2 Beets (nitric-oxide to oxygenate the blood)
- 2 Pears
- 1" piece of ginger (anti-inflammatory)
- 1 Handful Of Spinach (strong bones)
- 1 cucumber (super hydration)

PRE-WORKOUT ENERGY BLAST JUICE

Get all the energy you need for your intense workouts with this refreshing blend.

Ingredients:

- 3 Beets
- 2 Large Carrots
- 2 Green Apples
- 2" Piece of Fresh Ginger
- 1/4 Lemon
- 1/4 Lime

IRON INFUSION JUICE

This juice is loaded with healthy iron rich vegetables for healthy production of hemoglobin, healthy red blood cells, and fighting fatigue.

Ingredients:

- 1 Apple
- 1 Orange
- 6 to 7 Spinach leaves
- 1/2 Beet Including The Leafy Tops

GREEN IRON POWER JUICE

Another iron rich blend, with super healthy greens and ginger that fights inflammation.

Ingredients:

- 35 Spinach Leaves
- 25 Sprigs Of Fresh Mint
- 15 Sprigs Of Fresh Coriander
- 1/2 Lime
- 1" Piece Of Ginger
- 1/2 Lemon

VITAMIN D INFUSION JUICE

Get your vitamin D fix from this blend.

Ingredients:

- Handful Of Kale leaves
- Handful Of Spinach Leaves
- 1 kohlrabi
- 1 Cucumber
- 1 Mango
- 1 Grapefruit
- 1 Peach

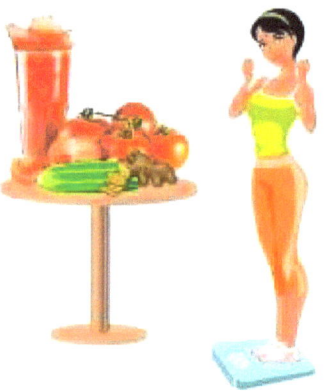

Conclusion

Juicing is a quick and convenient way to get all those micronutrients you need. You can make enough juice for 2 or 3 days and take it along to the gym in a thermos or have it within easy reach in your fridge when you come back from a run.

Its convenience can't be beat, eliminating the time and inclination to chew up to 3 or 4 bowls of vegetables every day.

Juicing is something that helps you to reach your goals. It is enjoyable - most people love it - and you can experiment as much as you want.

50 Tips to Juice Like a Pro

It's Time to Boost Your Health & Wellbeing

The plain and simple truth is that juicing provides essential vitamins, minerals, enzymes and other key nutrients, all of which support maximum wellness to prevent illness and combat stress.

50 Tips To Juice Like A Pro

1. Make a commitment to juicing and stick to it, this can be tricky if you are not used to the practice but with time, dedication and regular use it can become so deeply embedded that it will simply be something you won't want to live without. It can take several weeks to form a solid juicing habit, so stick with it and make sure to juice regularly.

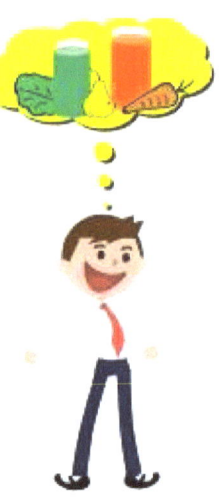

2. Create a juicing schedule. Make plans depending on how much your juicer can juice at one time, how much prep is necessary for produce, and how much time you can dedicate each day or every other day to be sure that you have fresh juice available at all times.

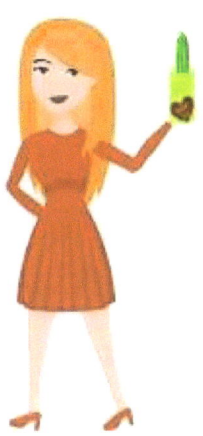

3. Stick with a regular juicing schedule to support the habit. Studies show that consumption of large doses of specific vitamins, minerals, and enzymes can aid in the prevention and management of symptoms associated with heart disease, cancer, and strokes and can strengthen immunity against colds and flu, increase bone density and improve the condition of the skin. We know that studies have shown that it is recommended that we consume six to eight servings of vegetables and fruits daily. This can be challenging for many people, juicing ensures that you reach the recommended daily intake for vegetables in a convenient manner.

4. Buy a quality juicer - many vegetables, like beets and carrots, are actually quite difficult to pulverize properly, and cheap juicers will not do the job. Buying a juicer that is powerful enough to pulverize efficiently and rapidly is one of the keys to buying a great juicer. If you plan to juice a lot of hard vegetables, your best choice is a centrifugal juicer.

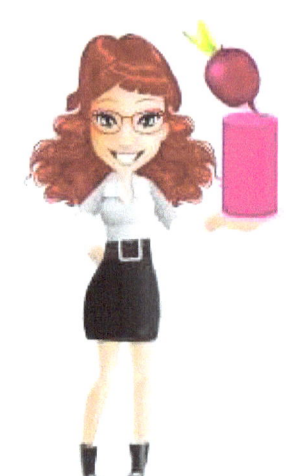

5. If you plan to juice mostly greens, then consider a masticating juicer that is great for greens and also supplies a high juice yield.

6. Consider the size of the mixing container. If you go too small, you'll only be able to juice a little at a time, so make sure you invest in a unit that has the capacity for your juicing needs. This is especially important for large families.

7. Keep a produce shopping list to stay organized and have all the ingredients you need at hand when you want to juice.

8. If you plan to juice in the morning then prep your produce as needed the night before. This is especially useful when your mornings are rushed or time limited.

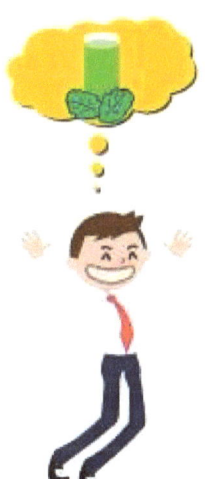

9. Always wash produce thoroughly to eliminate all dirt particles, and some of the pesticides when not buying organic produce. This is especially important with leafy greens where dirt hides between the leaves.

10. Line your juicer's pulp basket with a plastic bag for easy clean up.

11. Juice every day to build a healthy habit. When daily juicing is not possible, you can store juice in the fridge in an airtight container for up to 3 days.

12. Juice vegetables that you do not normally eat. Every vegetable provides a different benefit to the body but everyone is different in terms of what vegetables they enjoy eating, and so they skip those they don't like due to either taste, smell or texture. Juicing these allows you to obtain benefits from vegetables that you would not ordinarily consume, and since you can mask their taste with fruit, lemons, ginger and other enhancers getting these nutrients becomes much less of a burden.

13. Consider sugar content of fruits when you juice, as some have so much sugar they should be consumed in moderation or avoided altogether, especially for those who need to avoid spikes in blood sugar levels (diabetics), those with weight issues, and definitely those who are juicing for weight loss.

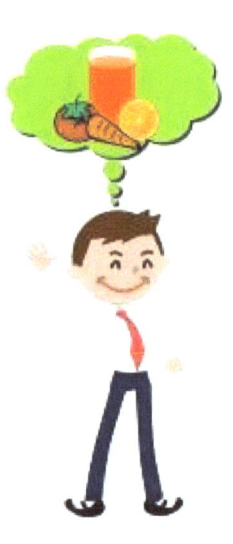

14. Taste as you go and adjust accordingly, just as you would during cooking.

15. Consuming juices first thing in the morning or at any time when your stomach is empty will optimize the rate at which the vitamins, minerals, antioxidants, and enzymes are absorbed and used by the body. It also gives you a great energy boost to kick-start your day with the drive you need. Additionally, consuming raw fruit and vegetables provides an intensive boost of vitamins and enzymes, which are directed straight to the blood stream. This means that your digestive system does not need to process the fruit and vegetables as they would if you were to consume them whole.

16. Juice high water vegetables, like cucumbers and broccoli. People often struggle with reaching the recommended daily intake of water. With six to eight glasses being the goal, some find it difficult to reach this intake. Many juicing combinations incorporate an element of water as the basis 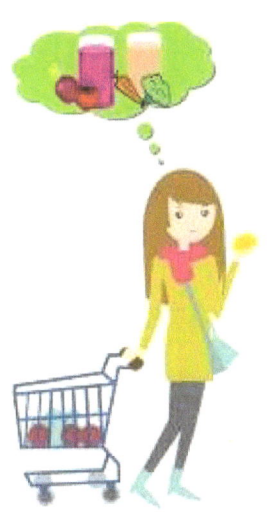 for the recipe, and indeed many vegetables and fruits have a high water concentration, meaning that you are extracting water during the juicing process.

Juicing provides a great strategy for increasing your water intake each day to hydrate your body.

17. Make sure to juice vegetables with fruit. If you only consume fruit based juices, your intake of sugar and calories will be unnecessarily high. By integrating vegetable juicing into your daily diet, you will be able to optimize the volume of vitamins, minerals, antioxidants, and enzymes being absorbed by your body.

18. Make sure that you follow the 80/20 rule when it comes to the ratio of vegetables to fruit. 80% vegetables that will give you the immunity, wellness, and energy boost you need and 20% fruit for more nutrients and taste. So, add an apple to give some sweetness or an orange if you crave some zesty citrus flavor.

19. Make sure that you include one or two root vegetables in your juicing combination. By adding in a carrot or beet into your recipe, you will be able to give the juice an intense boost of antioxidants, while also gaining a sweet but earthy flavor, which makes it more palatable when drinking.

20. To optimize the nutritional properties of your juice you need to ensure that you include a minimum of at least, one leafy green vegetable such as kale, broccoli, or chard, which will give you an enormous amount of unique nutrients.

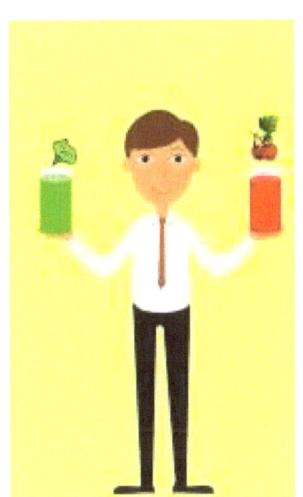

21. High water content vegetables such as a cucumbers or celery will assist in diffusing the very (and sometimes overpowering) flavors of kale, broccoli, or chard, which help to ensure that the juice you prepare is easy to drink.

22. Add some kind of garnish to not only provide a concentrated and intensive vitamin boost but also to make the juice really tasty. Great options include, ginger, lemons, limes or mint.

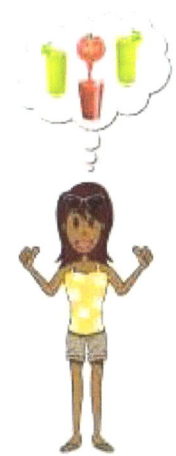

23. Re-juice any still wet pulp to get the most bang for your juicing buck.

24. Juice to improve the aging process - as we age our ability to digest what we need can become impaired as our organs work less optimally. By preparing food in this liquid and raw form, it becomes "pre-digested" which means that the body can absorb the vitamins, minerals, antioxidants and enzymes quickly and most efficiently.

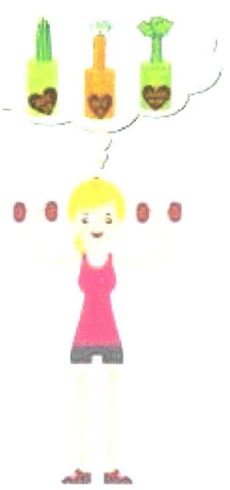

25. Juicing fruit alone greatly increases your sugar intake, which can lead to weight gain and erratic blood sugar spikes that actually stimulate hunger, negating the positive benefits that juicing offers.

26. Include lots of vegetables in your juicing to benefit from chlorophyll, which is a compound that acts as the life force within the plant. This compound also offers significant beneficial properties for humans.

27. Consumed raw as part of a juicing regime, the chlorophyll is digested straight into your bloodstream meaning that you are getting all of the benefits that the vegetables have to offer. Wheatgrass has the highest amount of chlorophyll.

28. Drink more green juice. Green juice is juice made mostly from dark leafy greens, such as kale, broccoli, and spinach, but can also include celery, cabbage, broccoli, and apples. Green juice is your best choice in a highly nutrient rich and low sugar drink.

29. For some, the perception that green colored juice looks bad and therefore tastes bad can interfere with the healthy practice of juicing. You can get past your perceived dislike for the color of the juice by adding in some red berries or orange carrots that will improve the color and taste to get a boost of vitamins, minerals, antioxidants and enzymes that you need to optimize your mental and physical health and wellbeing.

30. To help you become acclimated to the taste of vegetable juice, ease yourself into the taste of green vegetable-based juices so that you aren't immediately repelled and become turned off juicing forever. Start with mild-tasting vegetables such as celery and cucumbers. As you start to build your juicing palette, you can start to incorporate lettuce, kale, spinach, parsley, or cilantro.

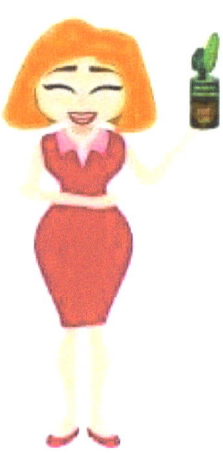

31. To counteract that bitterness of vegetable and green juices, you can add in elements of lemon or lime, grapefruits, cranberries or ginger, each of which have excellent properties that are associated with health and wellbeing.

32. Continue to eat whole vegetables and fruits even while juicing as they produce important insoluble fiber that your body needs.

33. It is best to consume juice on an empty stomach. This will give your body an optimum energy boost and allow for optimal digestion of all of the vitamins, minerals, antioxidants and enzymes that you need to go about your day.

34. Engage the whole family in juicing, as this is a great way to increase vegetable intake in young kids who hate eating them to make sure they benefit from the regular consumption of vitamins, minerals, antioxidants, and enzymes.

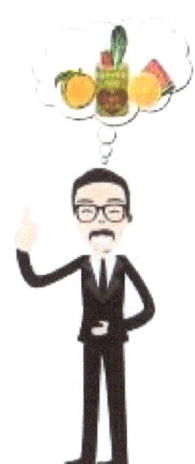

35. Collect juicing recipes, but also create your own blends to find combinations that please your palate and allow you to remain positive about your new habit.

36. To improve the health and vitality of your skin try combining cucumbers and a small apple (for taste).

37. To fight aging, choose a juicing combination that includes water/milk/aloe-vera juice, blueberries, strawberries, kale, and beetroot.

38. To enhance your libido you can combine coconut water, celery, banana, ginger, basil, and figs.

39. To give yourself an energy boost juice a combination that includes cucumbers, celery, kale, spinach, parsley, lemon and ginger.

40. To satisfy your sweet tooth juice a combination that includes apples, celery, and stir in a little cinnamon.

41. To boost your immune system and prevent the cold and flu, juice blends that include beetroot, carrots, celery, broccoli, garlic, ginger, lemon, and cayenne pepper.

42. If you are overworked or feeling the effects of stress in your life, prepare a stress relief juice with spinach, broccoli, celery, and carrots.

43. If you want to improve your gut health and digestion, boost your intake of papain, which is an enzyme found in papaya that helps digest proteins. Try a juice that includes papaya, kale, cabbage, ginger, and lemon.

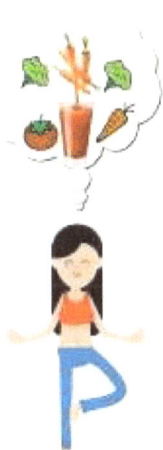

44. Juice organic produce - Use only organic vegetables to avoid toxins, and to increase the nutritional value of your produce and healthy enzyme intake.

45. Enhance your juices with ground nuts and seeds and protein powders.
Adding protein powder to your juice makes for a great meal replacement juice.

46. Beware of long term juice cleanses, and make sure to ask your doctor before starting any sort of juice fast.

47. Engage your kids in the juicing process. Let them pick out their own ingredients to get them excited about fruits and vegetables.

48. Buy an airtight container so you can refrigerate your juice and also take it with you to work, the gym or while running errands.

49. If you have an adversity to the taste of vegetable juice, don't worry, for many it is an acquired taste. Once your body starts to feel the health benefits you'll be hooked.

50. Balance high yield produce like celery, tomatoes, apples, and cucumbers, with a low yield vegetable like kale to get more juice in your glass.

Other Health and Fitness Books by This Author

If you would like to read more about Senior Health and Fitness, here is a list of the <u>titles, CreateSpace links and descriptions:</u>

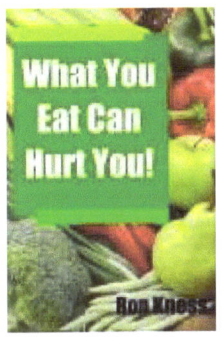

[What You Eat Can Hurt You](https://www.createspace.com/4963196)

https://www.createspace.com/4963196

Do you know that certain foods increase your risk for inflammation, disease and illness? It's true! And certain foods can help cure and heal you if you do get sick. Knowing which foods to eat and which ones to avoid empowers you to manage your own health.

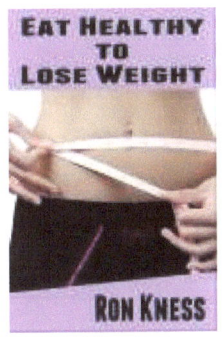

[Eat Healthy to Lose Weight](https://www.createspace.com/4962939)

https://www.createspace.com/4962939

As you read through our book, we show you which foods you should and should not be eating to reach your weight loss goal, along with discussing how to maintain your weight loss and stay within a few pounds of your goal weight. Banish the weight you keep gaining back each time by learning how to live a healthy lifestyle.

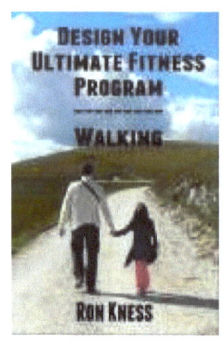

Design Your Ultimate Fitness Program - Walking

https://www.createspace.com/5252272

In my book Design Your Ultimate Fitness Program – Walking, we discuss the considerations that need to be made when designing a custom walking program, along with:
• Equipment needed
• Wearable technology you can use to track your walking
• And how to make walking more challenging

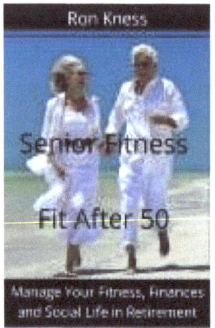

Senior Fitness – Fit After 50: Learn How to Manage Your Fitness, Finances and Social Life in Retirement

https://www.createspace.com/5474751

Inside you will discover answers to your most pressing questions:
• What do I need to know about downsizing my home?
• What are the best tips for staying healthy as you approach your 50's?
• When should I start planning for retirement?
• I am worried about being lonely once I retire, do others feel the same?
• Is it worthwhile to carry two homes during retirement?
And more…

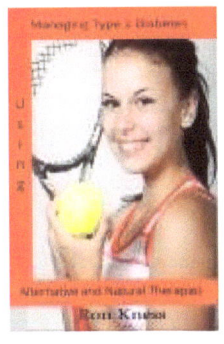

Managing Type 2 Diabetes Using Alternative And Natural Therapies

https://www.createspace.com/5401244

While Type 2 diabetes can be managed medically, there are many alternative natural and holistic methods of therapy and treatment that can further enhance quality of life and minimize the effects of this disease. In this book, I discuss 12 different types, including yoga, reflexology and acupuncture to name just three.

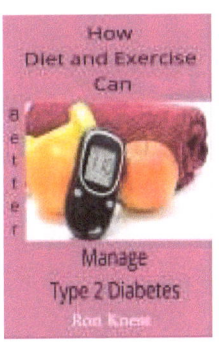

How Diet and Exercise Can Better Manage Type 2 Diabetes

https://www.createspace.com/5404845

Of the different types of diabetes, only Type 2 can be reversed. In my book How Diet and Exercise Can Better Manage Type 2 Diabetes, we reveal the three things you can do to best manage your disease, including:
• Diet
• Exercise
• Weight management

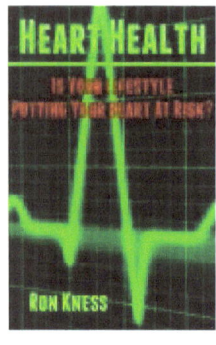

[Heart Health: Is Your Lifestyle Putting Your Heart at Risk?](#)

https://www.createspace.com/5464020

In my ebook Is Your Lifestyle Putting Your Heart At Risk? we discuss the six greatest risks to your heart and the lifestyle changes you can make to mitigate them.

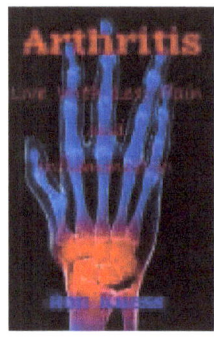

[Arthritis – Live Wth Less Pain and Inflammation: Tips and Techniques You Can Use to Lessen the Pain and Inflammation](#)

https://www.createspace.com/5457441

Discover Simple Tips & Information That Will Help Reduce The Painful Symptoms Of Arthritis!

You learn things like:
• Simple and effective information that will help you manage the pain and inflammation that comes along with arthritis, so that you can live an active, full life without debilitating pain.
• The different types of arthritis, their symptoms and how to alleviate their painful side effects.
• The pros and cons of over-the-counter arthritis medications, plus simple tips that will help you know how to choose the right supplements.
• Free, yet effective ways to get relief from arthritis pain and inflammation, so you don't have to suffer anymore.

The effects arthritis can have significant impact on your physical and mental well-being, but this books shows you how to overcome its painful symptoms and live life relatively pain free.

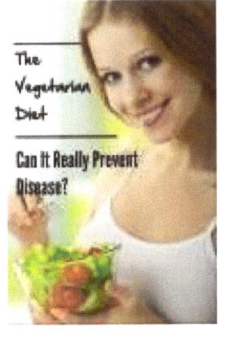

The Vegetarian Diet – Can It Really Prevent Disease?

https://www.createspace.com/5519874

Is a vegetarian diet right for you? Multiple studies have shown over and over that a vegetarian diet goes along way in preventing certain chronic diseases, such as:

• Heart Disease
• Cancer
• Diverticulitis
• Type 2 Diabetes
• Hypertension
• Obesity
• Kidney Failure

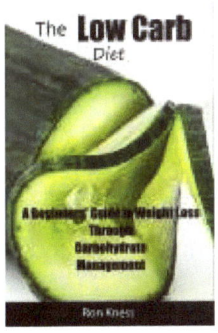

The Low Carb Diet: A Beginner's Guide to Weight Loss Through Carbohydrate Management

https://www.createspace.com/5416348

In my book "The Low-Carb Diet – A Beginners' Guide to Weight Loss Through Carbohydrate Management", I reveal a successful method of losing weight based in part on the amount and type of carbohydrates you consume.

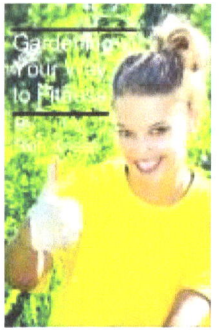

Gardening Your Way to Fitness: The Fun Way to Get Fit and Provide Beauty and Healthful Bounty for Your Family

https://www.createspace.com/5459564

The gym is a great place to stay fit during the colder seasons, but once the temperature turns warmer you want to spend more time outside. Plus, you'll have the benefit of fresh wholesome produce to enjoy by growing vegetables in your backyard garden.

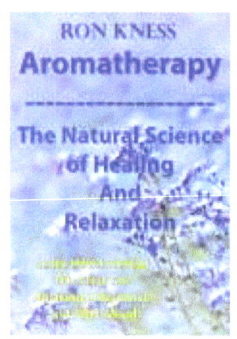

Aromatherapy - The Science of Healing and Relaxation: Learn How Essential Oils Elicit The Relaxation Response And Alter Mood

https://www.createspace.com/5714434

In my book Aromatherapy – The Science of Healing and Relaxation, we reveal the natural holistics methods you can use to heal the body from certain medical issues and to relive stress through relaxation. In particular we talk about:
• Aromatherapy - what it is and how it works
• Essential Oils – how the effects of certain aromas differs from others
• Recipes – how to make your own essential oil combinations

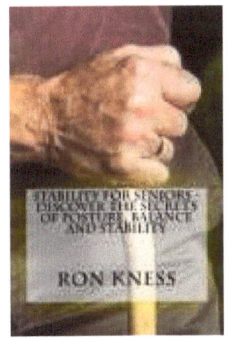

Stability for Seniors: Discover the Secrets of Posture, Balance and Stability

https://www.createspace.com/6096479

Many people sacrifice their health in pursuit of their career. They are so busy making a living that they neglect to make a life. The excuse that they do not have time to exercise is tossed about so frequently that they end up letting their health and fitness slide.

If you are not regularly active, you will have muscular atrophy over time. Your flexibility will decrease. Your core strength will diminish. As time progresses, you will be less limber and more rigid.

This is exactly how people age poorly. It's a process that has snowballed over time.

Only with regular exercise and a healthy diet can you have a body that is fit and has the ability to almost reverse aging.

If you have neglected your health for years and life seems to be a chore now because you can't get around without assistance, do not feel dejected.

You can remedy the situation. You can restore the strength, balance and stamina that you have lost. It is never too late to become what you might have been.

This guide will show you exactly what you need to do to restore your balance, strengthen your core and give you the ability to live life to its fullest. Read how …

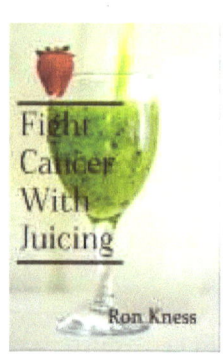

Fight Cancer With Juicing

https://www.createspace.com/6155567

Juicing is a healthy practice that has allowed millions of people to boost their nutrition. Juicing fruits and vegetables provides you important antioxidants, which scavenge for oxygen free radicals that can damage cellular structures, including DNA. When DNA is damaged, it can result in mutations that lead to cancer.

Well-balanced nutrition from a variety of healthy whole foods helps support and maintain on-going good health, and experts agree that nutrition plays a key role in preventing chronic and terminal illness.

Juicing is practiced by millions around the world and it is an easy and convenient way to get plant nutrition into the body to do its magic.

When juicing is done right, that is when the majority of your juice blends is comprised of vegetables and very low sugar fruit, you can easily boost your nutritional intake thereby improving your health and lower your risks for cancer.

About the Author

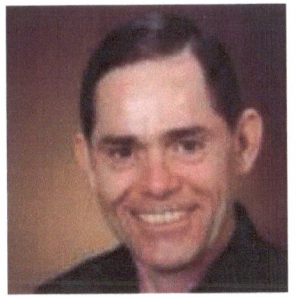

I grew up in Central Minnesota, where my parents own and operated a fishing resort. Once out of high school I tried a couple of semesters of college, only to quit halfway through the Spring term; I decided at that time that college wasn't for me.

Then I decided to follow my father's previous occupation as an auto mechanic. I graduated from a two-year of vocational training course and worked as a mechanic. While in vocational training, I decided to join the National Guard where I eventually ended up working full-time for 32 years.

So how does all of this relate to writing? In one of my leadership schools, the instructor, who was an English teacher at a juvenile detention center, presented writing to me in a whole new way - a way that started to develop my interest in working with words.

Fast forward about 40 years and I now have over 50 books listed on Amazon for Kindle and CreateSpace.

www.ingramcontent.com/pod-product-compliance
Lightning Source LLC
Chambersburg PA
CBHW050822290526
45792CB00001B/227